the **Handbag** book of **Inspirations**

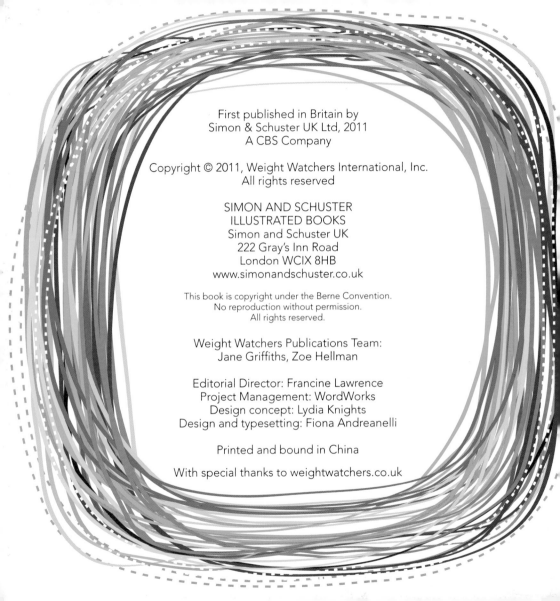

First published in Britain by
Simon & Schuster UK Ltd, 2011
A CBS Company

SIMON AND SCHUSTER
ILLUSTRATED BOOKS
Simon and Schuster UK
222 Gray's Inn Road
London WCIX 8HB
www.simonandschuster.co.uk

Weight Watchers Publications Team:
Jane Griffiths, Zoe Hellman

Editorial Director: Francine Lawrence
Project Management: WordWorks
Design concept: Lydia Knights
Design and typesetting: Fiona Andreanelli

Printed and bound in China

With special thanks to weightwatchers.co.uk

the **Handbag** book of **Inspirations**

Your essential guide to healthy living

⟲WeightWatchers®

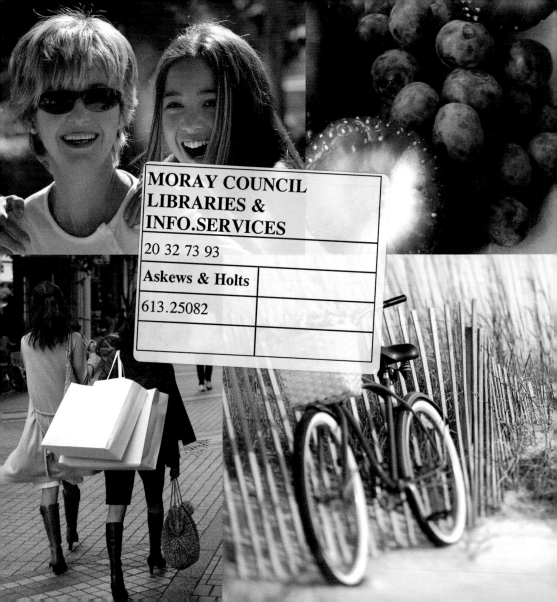

MORAY COUNCIL
LIBRARIES &
INFO.SERVICES

20 32 73 93	
Askews & Holts	
613.25082	

Contents

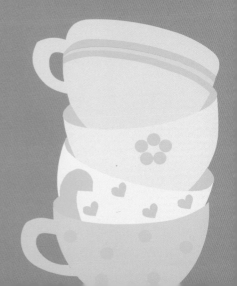

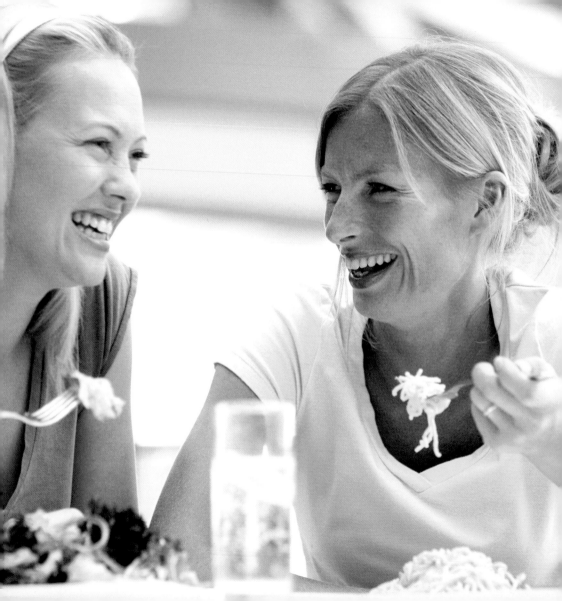

introduction

The Handbag Book of Inspirations is full of advice and affirmations for every woman who aspires to a healthy lifestyle and wants to enjoy life to the fullest, as she pursues her weight loss goals.

Keep this little book in your handbag, take it wherever you go and reach for it whenever you need a boost. **Discover great ways to stay motivated** or simply be inspired by a beautiful image or a word of wisdom to enjoy a moment of calm.

Enjoy parties and stay on track, eat out at restaurants and feel in control or relax on holiday and return feeling renewed and refreshed, instead of guilty and defeated. Whether you're sitting at your desk, chilling out after a long day or looking for the perfect pair of jeans on a shopping trip with friends, you'll find ideas for how to live a healthy, happy life. Make the most of beauty and relaxation tips too and look and feel **more confident**, **more beautiful**, **more radiant**.

Whatever you do, wherever you go, **be inspired** to embrace and enjoy the benefits of healthy living.

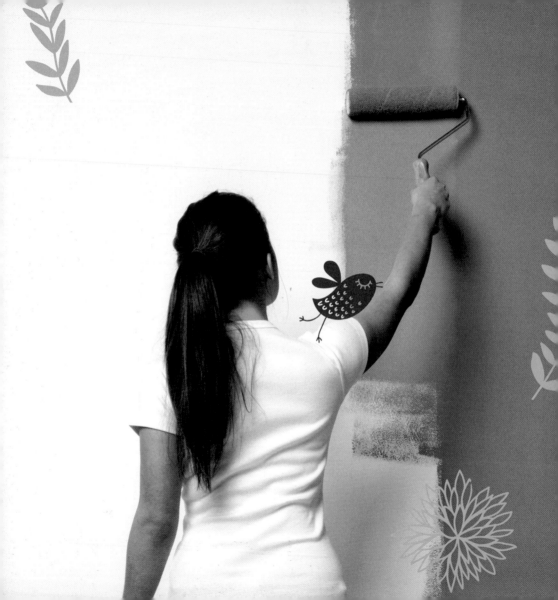

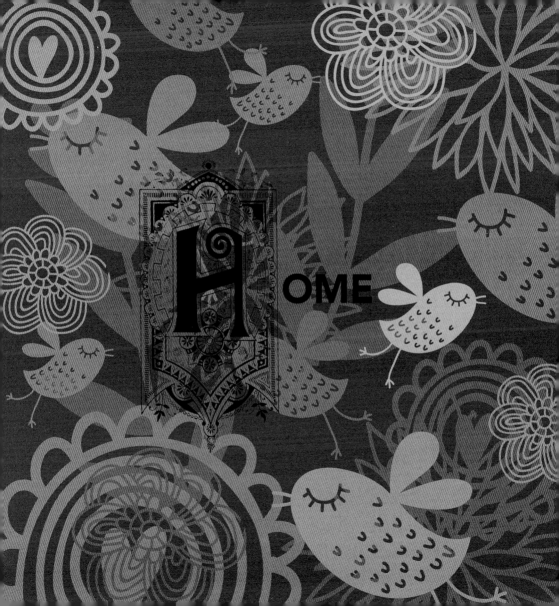

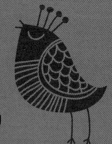

emotional eating

problem... some people get into the habit of using food for comfort

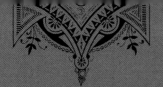

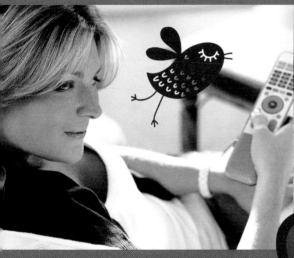

solution... think about why you are eating and name that feeling

When the habit to reach for food kicks in, opt for snacks that take time to prepare such as pistachios in the shell or fruit you need to peel or cut up. By the time you've finished preparing and eating them, your emotions may well be on the upswing.

01 Identify the times you tend to comfort eat. **02 Think** about why you want to eat. Are you unhappy, tired, worried? **03 Try** to find other ways to deal with your emotions and avoid the snacking urge.

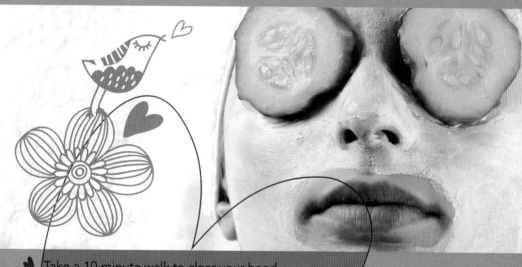

- Take a 10 minute walk to clear your head.
- Relax in a bubble bath with scented oils.
- Dip into your favourite magazine.
- Call a friend you haven't spoken to for ages.
- And if you still need to snack, why not have some fruit handy to eat?

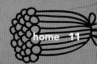

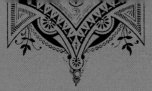

in your kitchen

fast food at home

Quick and easy, not fried and greasy; enjoy a home-made '**takeaway**'.

Burgers Make your own burgers with lean beef mince, onions and seasonings. Grill them slowly and use tasty relishes and salsas instead of mayo sauces.

Crispy coated fish Dip fish fillets into beaten egg white, seasoned with garlic, mustard powder or chopped herbs and then dip them into crushed cornflakes, oatmeal or breadcrumbs. Bake for about 20 minutes until the topping is crisp.

Chunky chips Peel some big potatoes and cut lengthways into wedges. Par-boil for just a minute or two, drain and spritz with spray oil. Bake for 30 minutes until brown and crispy.

Quick chicken Remove the skin from the chicken portions, roll each piece in a mixture of breadcrumbs, chilli, black pepper and finely grated Parmesan cheese. Bake in a hot oven for around 45 minutes.

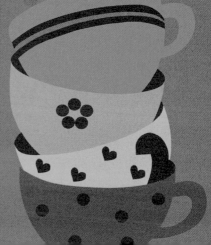

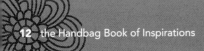

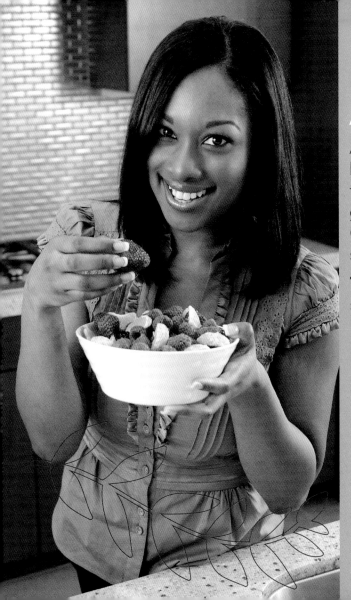

AFTER WORK FIX

After work, you're often hungry but dinner isn't for a few hours. **Don't give in to temptation**. Grab a healthy and satisfying snack.

TRY a handful of nuts, seeds and dried fruit, a pot of low fat yogurt, a cracker or veggies with low fat houmous. You could enjoy a small bowl of cereal, grab a banana or try a couple of slices of wafer thin ham and some cherry tomatoes.

get your life into SHAPE

Everyday activities can give your body a **fantastic workout** without the expense of joining a gym. Simply start small.

'Anything is better than nothing'
...make life's everyday activities work for you

Leg work View a cluttered floor as a chance to get some leg work in. Bend your knees when putting things away for a great leg workout.

Change your mindset Set yourself mini activity goals – use excuses like 'I have to go to the postbox' or 'I need to visit the cash machine' to enjoy some fresh air and do some walking.

TV workout Use the advert breaks during your favourite tv show for a great workout. Try to complete one set of 20 lunges, squats, crunches, arm circles or do as many push-ups as you can during each break.

Energize Play some lively music while you work – you'll sweep faster and scrub harder. Each time you pass a mirror, you can smile knowing that your efforts are whittling your waist while shining up your home.

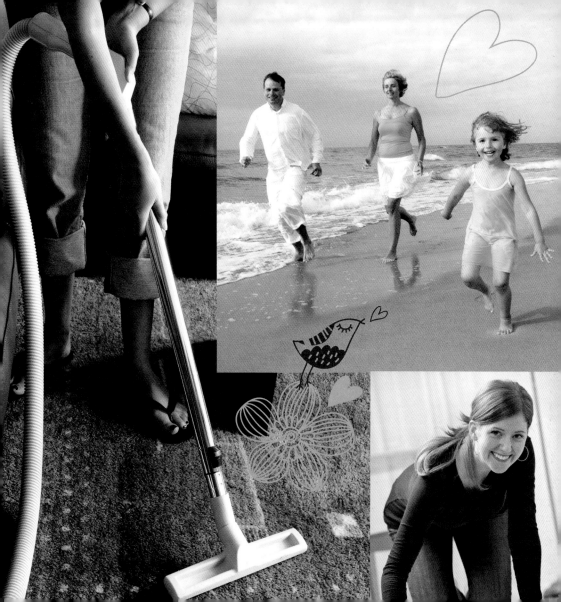

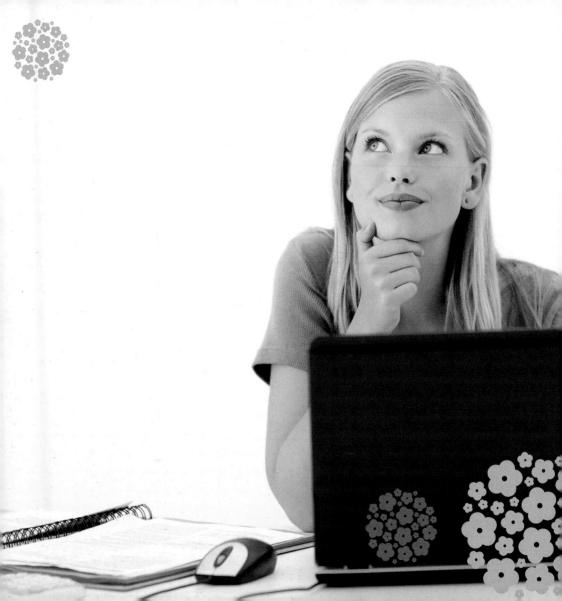

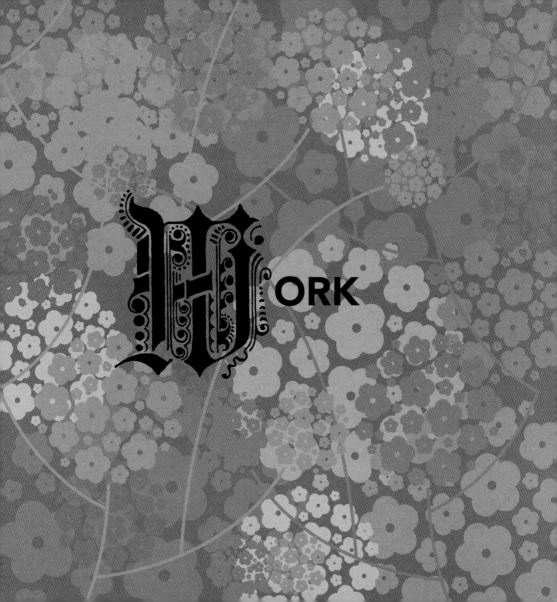

a quick lunch

problem... in a rush? Forgot to pack lunch?
At home and need to grab something quick between emails?

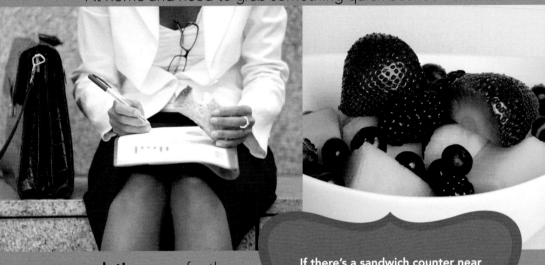

solution... go for the
healthy food choices

If there's a sandwich counter near
you, tell them what you want and
watch the sandwich being made
up in front of you.

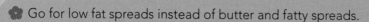

- Go for low fat spreads instead of butter and fatty spreads.
- Enjoy a strong-tasting cheese since you don't need as much.
- Bulk out a sandwich with lettuce, cucumber, tomatoes, cress, beetroot or any other salad item you fancy.
- Choose lean cuts of meat or cut the fat off.

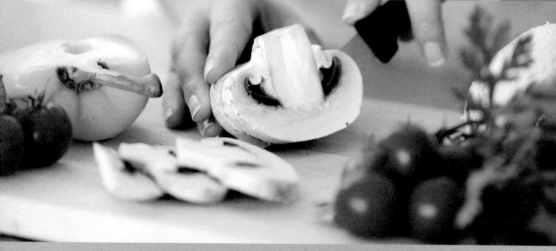

We all need **TREATS** to keep us going so stock up on healthy snacks, hiding them in desk drawers, handbags and briefcases.
01 A banana or apple **02** A Weight Watchers bar **03** Mini boxes of raisins
04 A bag of unsalted nuts with mixed fruit **05** Pine nuts

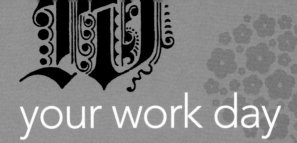

your work day

get up and go

Set your alarm clock for half an hour earlier and go for a walk, or do some indoor exercise at the gym. Prepare your gym bag and outfit the night before for a quick start.

park and walk

Park as far away as possible from the office, or get off a stop or two earlier, and walk the rest of the way. You can then walk back again after work.

socialize and exercise

Arrange to meet up with colleagues over the lunch hour. Have a walk and enjoy a good chat or gossip – and yes, walking around the shops counts.

unwind

Why not ask your colleagues, or neighbours if you work at home, to split the cost of a masseuse to give you all a 15–20 minute neck and shoulder massage and unwind those tense muscles?

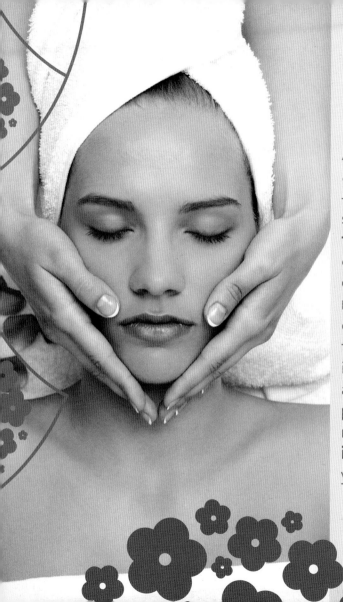

FIT IN A FACIAL

At lunchtime, stop by a cosmetics counter – you may find some hidden **free treats**. Many top cosmetic houses offer **complementary makeovers** by a qualified beautician, the price of which is offset against anything you may purchase from the range. Try on **new ideas** and update your make-up routine.

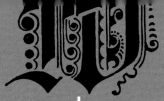

work out at work

How can I stay **active** and on track with **healthy habits** when I'm sitting behind a desk all day at work? Simple. Just build in **lots of small movements** – they really can make a big difference to your activity levels.

disguise exercise

To strengthen calf and abdominal muscles – and to help your posture – sit up straight and squeeze your stomach as you lift up your toes to tighten your calves. Work the calf muscles further and shape up your ankles by stretching your leg and pointing your toes forward and backwards 20 times, then make a circle with your feet and ankles 20 times on each foot.

stand up

When you pick up your phone, stand up to give your body a stretch. Try to keep any files you use in an overhead compartment so you need to stand up to reach them.

go the distance

Start using the toilets further away from your desk. Refill your water at a cooler on the other side of the office. It's a great opportunity to meet new colleagues, and no one will know your ulterior motive.

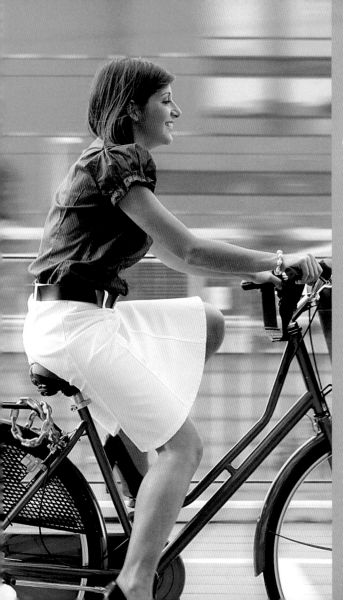

STRETCH
THEN SNACK

When you go to the kitchen to make tea, **do a lap or two around the office** before sitting down to enjoy it.

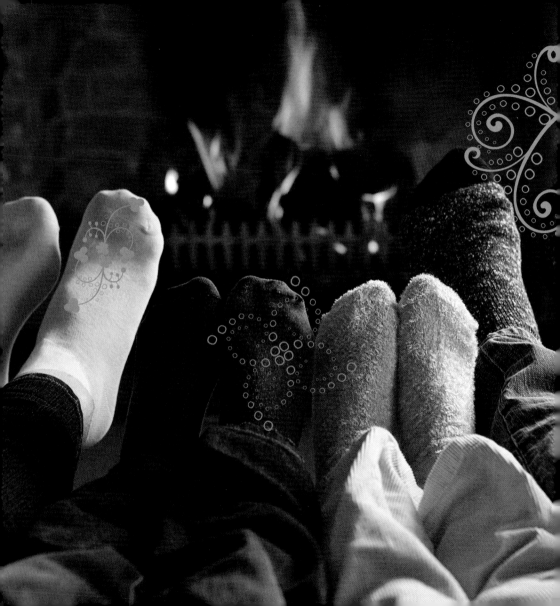

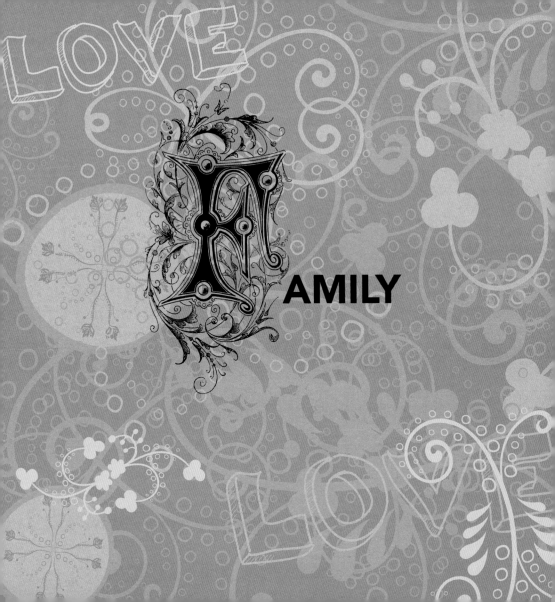

FAMILY

get the family on side

problem... do you need more support?

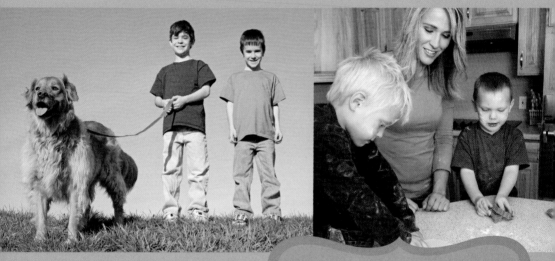

solution... turn the family on to healthy food tastes by letting them see how much you enjoy healthy food

Make your own cereal: Combine 30g of rolled oats, 1 sliced banana, 150g of low fat natural yogurt and 20g of chopped walnuts in a bowl. Keep it interesting and change the fruit and nut ingredients from day to day.

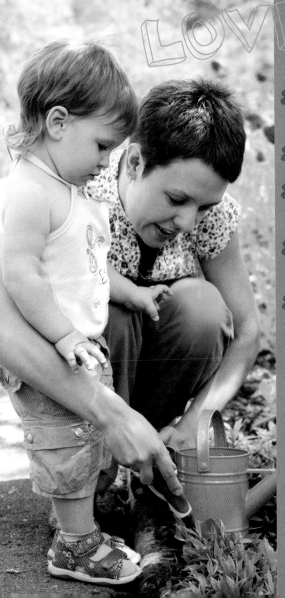

help the kids out

▶ **Stock the fridge** with wholesome, nutritious foods so that when teenagers raid it, they'll be enjoying healthy snacks.

▶ **Treat the kids** with home-made cakes, smoothies and dried fruit.

▶ **Buy fewer biscuits**, crisps, fizzy drinks and other snack foods. If it's not there, they won't eat it.

▶ **Try tasting sessions**, reward schemes, stickers and other prizes for younger children.

▶ **Teach your children** how to prepare easy, good-for-you snacks such as a ham salad sandwich.

win your partner over

01 Make your partner feel more included. Talk openly about what you want and how he or she can support you.
02 Think of ways to be together that don't involve food. Visit an exhibition or go to the cinema.
03 Find an activity you both enjoy and stay fit together by dancing, swimming, cycling or rowing.

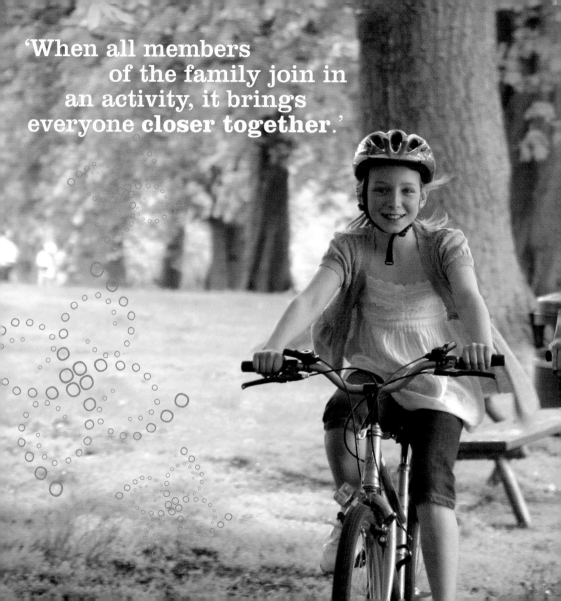

'When all members
     of the family join in
an activity, it brings
everyone **closer together**.'

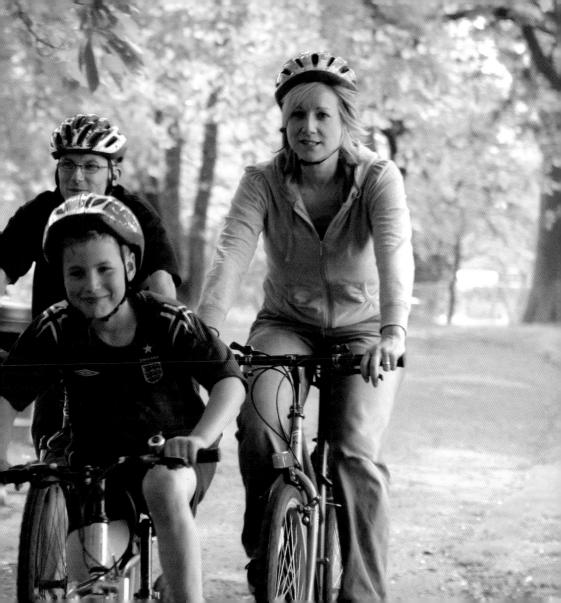

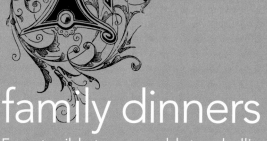

family dinners

From terrible two year olds to rebellious teenagers, there's **never a dull moment** bringing up children. It's a challenge so if you're looking for a strategy, **find some inspiration here**.

unwind together

Sit down to dinner together as often as you can. Children who eat family dinners are likely to eat more healthily and a relaxed dinner table can help older children to open up about what's going on in their lives.

encourage them

Believing in your children gives them confidence and a positive attitude towards their achievements.

keep it simple

Serve water with meals instead of soft drinks or fruit juice. A jug with a fun design and a new set of glasses can make all the difference. Add some ice and lemon too.

gently, gently

Introduce new foods by serving them alongside those that are familiar. That way they're less overwhelming and children may be more willing to give the new food a try.

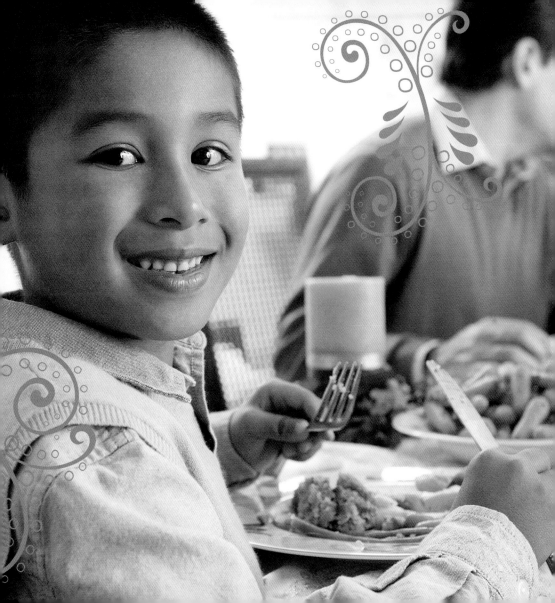

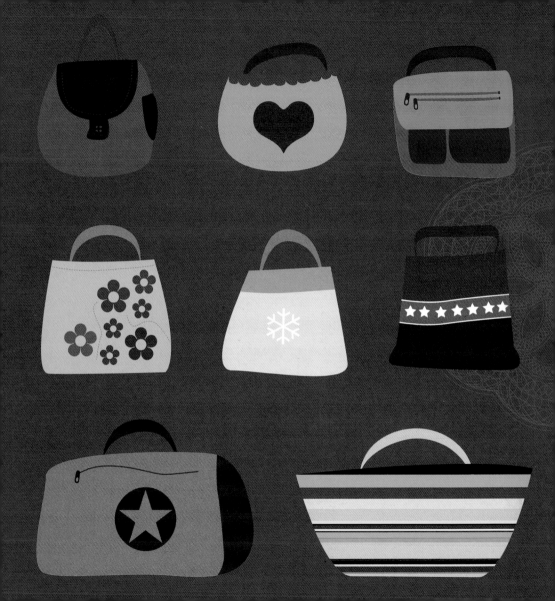

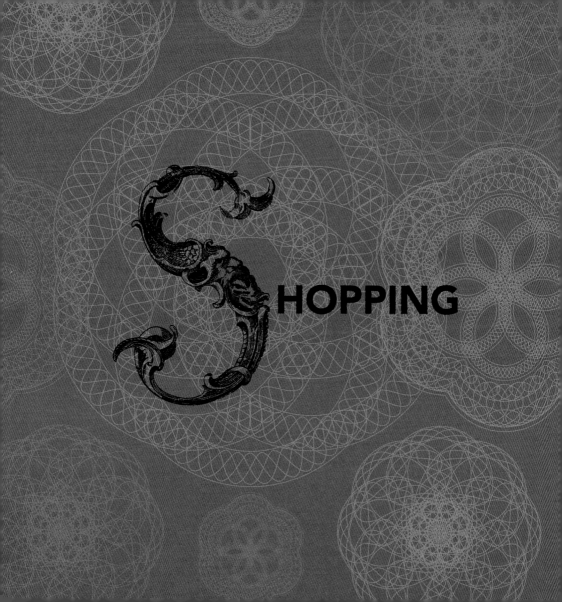

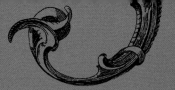

at the supermarket

problem... it's a challenge just to get through the weekly shop without buying more than you need

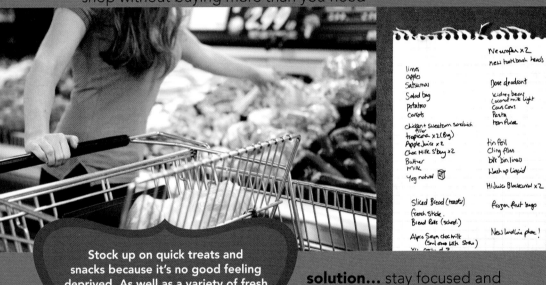

Nurofen x2
New toothbrush heads

limes
apples
Satsumas
Salad bag
potatoes
Carrots

Dove deodrant

Kidney beans
Coconut milk light
Cous Cous
Pasta
tom Puree

chicken + Sweetcorn sandwich filler
tropicana x 2 (Big)
Apple Juice x 2
Choc Milk S'bury x 2
Butter
Milk
Yog natural

tin foil
Cling film
blk bin liners
wash up Liquid

HiJuice Blackcurrant x 2

Sliced Bread (toasts)
French Stick
Bread Rolls (school)

Frozen fruit bags

New landline phone!

Alpro Soya choc milk
(Sml ones with Straw)

Stock up on quick treats and snacks because it's no good feeling deprived. As well as a variety of fresh fruits and vegetables, look for whole-grain cereal bars, baked crisps or mini rice cakes.

solution... stay focused and get through the aisles as swiftly and efficiently as possible

SHOP LOCALLY Instead of driving, why not **walk briskly** to the shops? Invest in a backpack or **give your arms some strength training** by carrying your shopping home – but make sure you don't overload yourself.

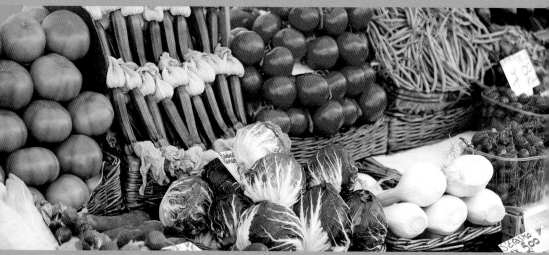

01 Plan ahead Write down your shopping list and stick to it. A good list really saves you time. **02 Quick shop** Organise your list according to the shop layout. **03 Eat before you go** If you're hungry, you may be more likely to reach for food that you don't actually need or want.

'You don't have to completely splash out on a new wardrobe. **Choosing one t-shirt** with a great cut that will emphasize your figure can make you feel better instantly.'

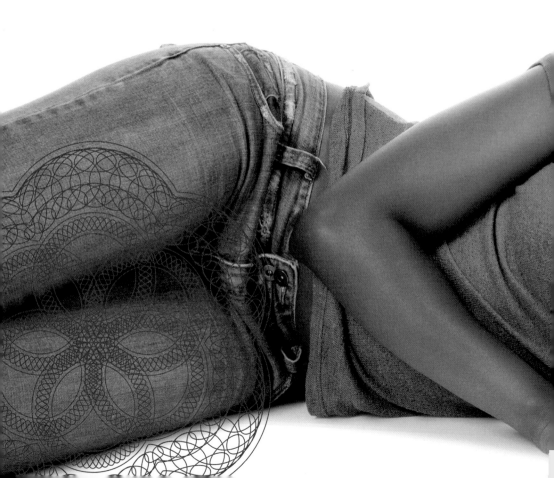

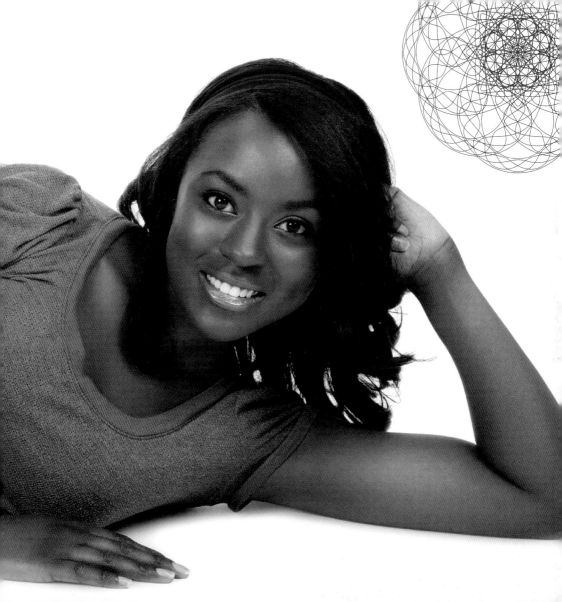

shopping for clothes

Let's face it, for most of us, the desire to **look fabulous** in our clothes is a major motivation for losing weight and buying new clothes is the **ultimate reward**. And you deserve it, so get the most out of your shopping trip with these tips.

shop when you feel good

Feeling positive about yourself, your body and your weight loss progress will help to prevent you from being overly self-critical when trying on styles. A good self-image goes a long way.

don't shop alone

Bring a friend, partner or sister with you – someone whose opinion you trust, and who makes you laugh. Then afterwards, you can enjoy a good chat together over a healthy lunch.

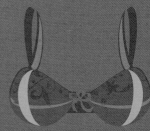

on the spot pick-me-up

Buy some lovely lingerie. Choose something that makes you feel special, not just what you think your partner might like – and start feeling good about yourself from the inside out.

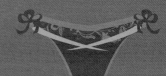

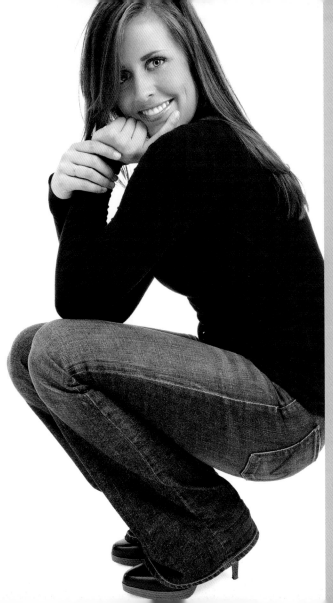

JEANS THAT FIT

Find jeans that make you **look good**. Choose a comfort stretch, with a lyrca blend. It allows for **SUPPORT**, without sacrificing **comfort**. If it suits you, a **flattering** boot cut can balance out the hip area. And a back pocket looks best, as long as it's not too small. If it's proportionate to the rest of the jean, it takes the eye away from the behind.

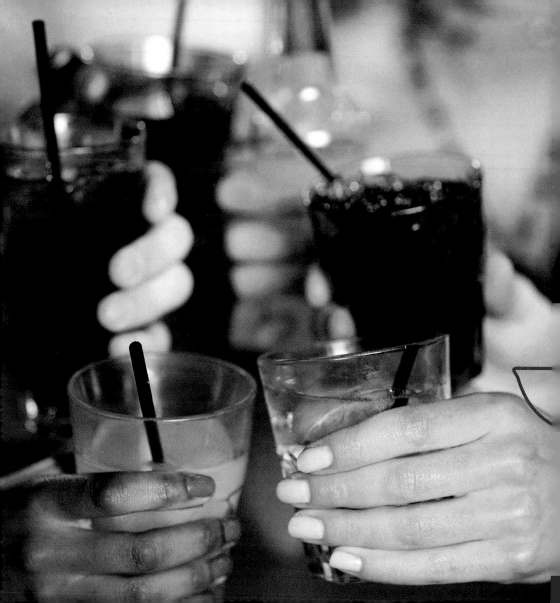

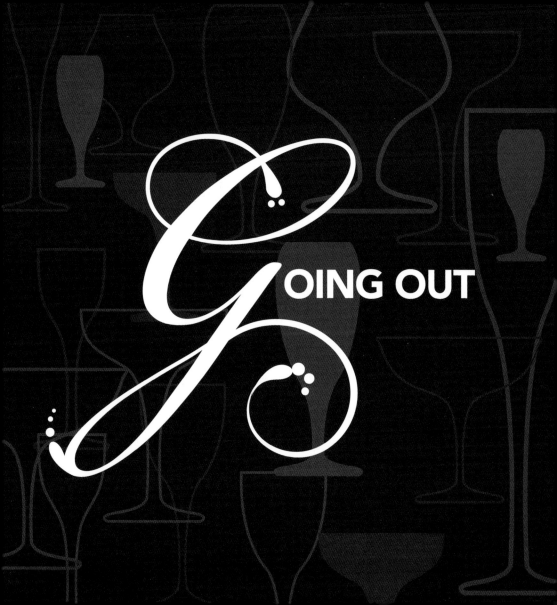

GOING OUT

parties

problem... you find it difficult to enjoy a party and stay on track with your weight loss too

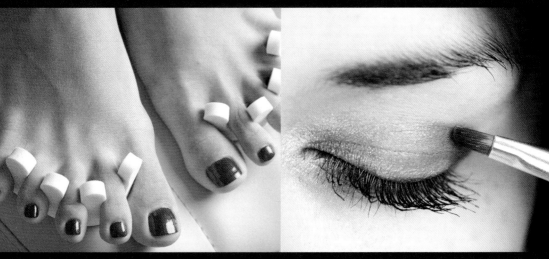

solution... it's fun to get ready for a party – choosing the dress, planning the make-up, deciding how to style your hair. Have a plan for the party food and drinks too and then **simply chill** and get into the **mood**

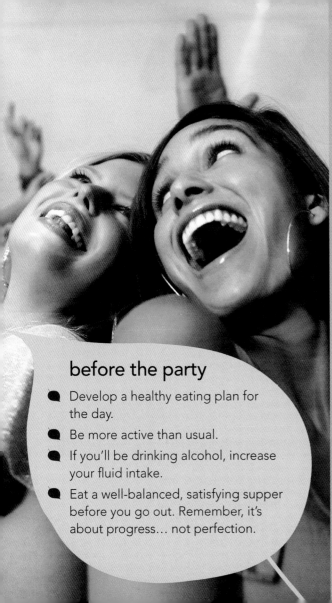

AT THE PARTY

Eat slowly Take real pleasure in eating every delicious mouthful.

Seating plan Don't sit near the food and drinks or at the bar. Walk through the crowd to get another drink or some food.

Go clubbing Get on to the dance floor. It burns calories and gives you great aerobic and cardiovascular exercise.

Socialize Walk from one group of people to the next to get a little more exercise and enjoy some new conversation. Once you've finished your meal, the more you can be distracted from the food, the better.

before the party

- Develop a healthy eating plan for the day.
- Be more active than usual.
- If you'll be drinking alcohol, increase your fluid intake.
- Eat a well-balanced, satisfying supper before you go out. Remember, it's about progress… not perfection.

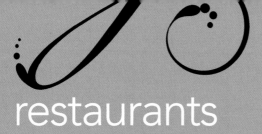
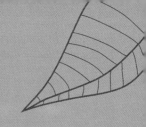

restaurants

Although we all **LOVE** to eat out, we may worry about going off track with our weight loss when we do. But you can **relax and leave your worries behind**. Whether you're going to a business lunch or enjoying dinner with friends...

...have a fab time with these tips...

Take charge Be the one to suggest a restaurant with health-conscious options such as a sushi restaurant.

Plan ahead Know what you want before you get there. Try to call ahead or look up the menu online.

The snack trick Keep a bag of apples or another healthy snack in your car, and have one before you go into the restaurant.

Just ask Most restaurants are happy to provide substitutions so don't be afraid to ask for help.

the art of BAMO

If things don't quite go the way you'd planned, remember to practise the art of BAMO: 'Breathe, Accept, Move On. '

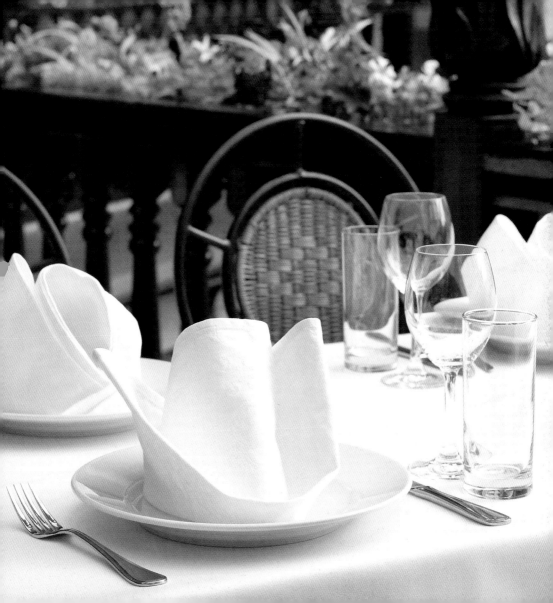

visiting family & friends

See occasions with family and friends as great **opportunities** to give yourself little goals to reach and then enjoy your success.

portion power

At a buffet, it can be all too easy to eat more than you need, or misjudge your portions, especially when you're surrounded by unfamiliar foods. Being aware of your portions can help you to stay in control so make sure you're portion savvy.

Spend a week measuring out your portions to get used to what a sensible serving looks like.

- Your fist is about the same size as one portion of fruit.
- Your thumb (tip to base) is the size of one portion of cheese.
- Your palm (minus fingers) equals a portion of meat, fish or poultry.
- Your cupped hand equals one portion of nuts or pretzels.

stay in control

If you're offered more food or drink at a family dinner, have an armoury of **useful responses** to resist temptation.

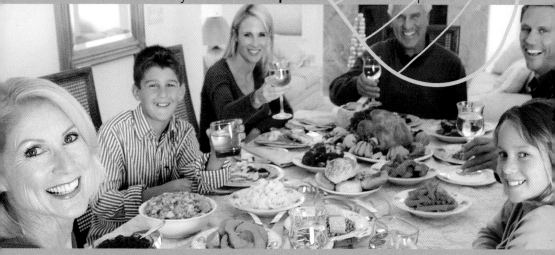

- Saying 'It was delicious but now I'm full thanks' **compliments** their cooking and leaves them **feeling good**.
- You could ask **how they made it** – this will take the focus away from you.
- **Offer to be the driver** at the party and stick to non-alcoholic drinks.

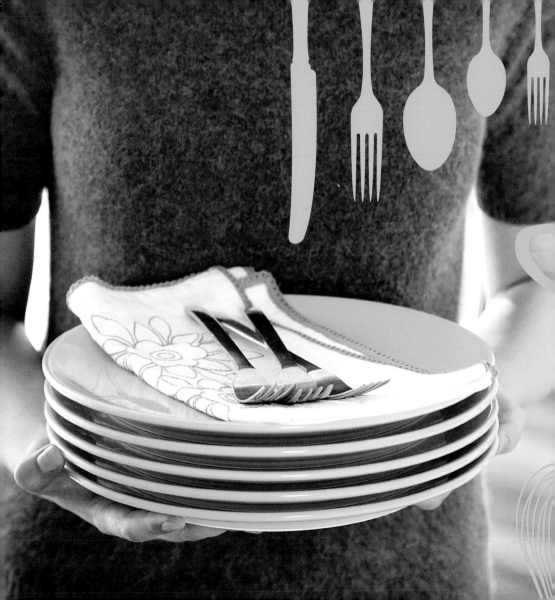

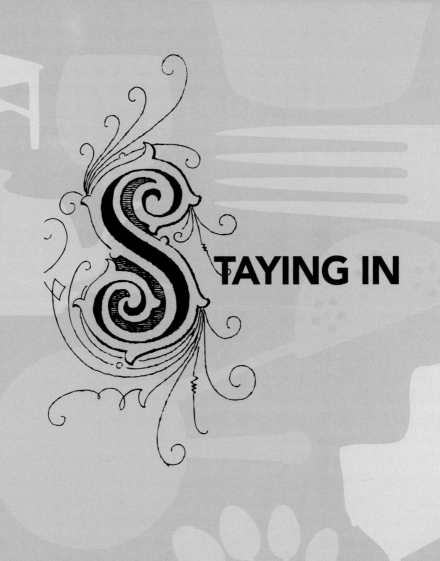

STAYING IN

celebrating at home

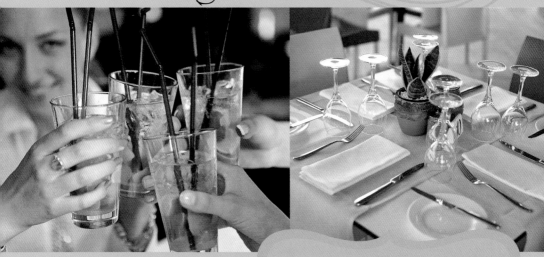

problem... celebrations always include food – along comes a birthday, anniversary or another event to lead you into temptation again

Make a list of accomplishments in every area of your life and look at the list often. Be your own cheerleader, become your own best friend. Celebrate your progress, and try not to obsess about setbacks.

solution... when you're entertaining at home, you're in control – so you can have a fabulous time, *your way*

It's your party Choose recipes from your Weight Watchers cookbooks or log on to weightwatchers.co.uk for some great recipe ideas and don't be surprised when everyone asks for the recipe.

Clever canapés Wow them with elegant canapés. Top miniature blinis with smoked salmon and a smidgen of reduced fat soured cream and dill or fill Little Gem lettuce leaves with houmous.

Go veggie Tuck into black bean burritos. Combine cooked, diced onions with canned black beans and a cooked rice mix then layer it down the centre of tortillas, top with salsa and low fat grated Cheddar cheese. Roll up and bake until heated through.

Sweeten the deal Fruits and fresh berries topped with low fat crème fraîche will satisfy a sweet tooth. For a cool finale, top a trio of sorbets with a sprig of mint or basil.

Low cal quaff Put out alcohol-free white or red grape juice or Weight Watchers Fruity White Wine on ice.

Jazz up juice Use fun ice cubes, sticks of celery and citrus zest. Experiment with colours.

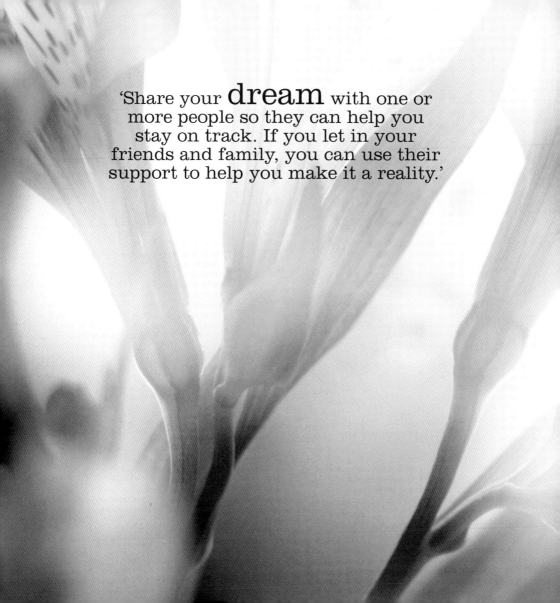

'Share your **dream** with one or more people so they can help you stay on track. If you let in your friends and family, you can use their support to help you make it a reality.'

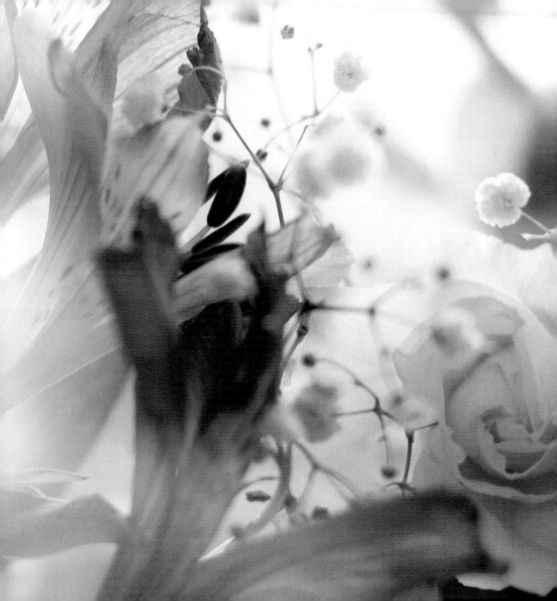

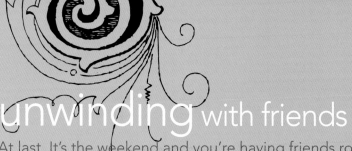

unwinding with friends

At last. It's the weekend and you're having friends round for an informal dinner or summer barbecue. Do you want to really chill out but not sabotage your plans to drop a few pounds? Get into the mood and **enjoy your company with confidence**.

...set the scene

Show off your fabulous sense of style. Little things make a real difference and your guests will appreciate them.

Instead of paper plates for a barbecue, lay out colourful and cheerful plastic ones.

Pick a fabulous tablecloth to create the mood.

Put out lots of candles and finish with vases of sunflowers.

...prepare to relax

If you're planning a buffet, remember that less is more. Prepare a few well-chosen dishes instead of lots of smaller options.

Aim to eat early in the evening, so you don't become ravenous and overeat or drink to try and fill the gap.

If you know you're prone to over-eating, have a low fat smoothie an hour or so before friends arrive.

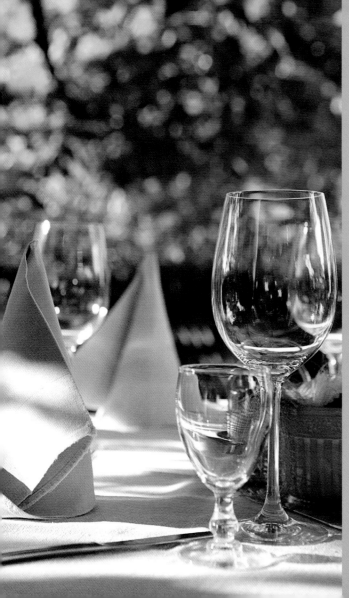

'Relax, have some laughs and enjoy catching up with your friends – focus on being with them and not on the food.'

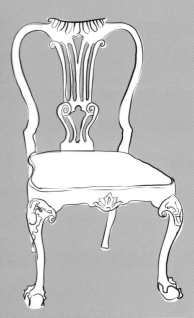

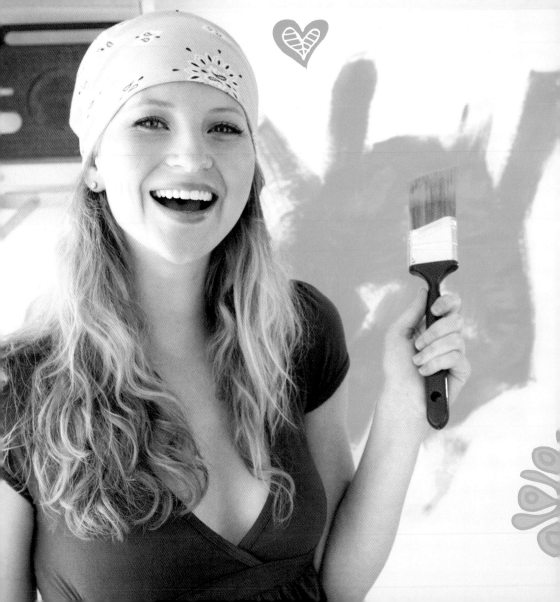

WHAT SHALL WE DO TODAY?

problem... life is so demanding, you don't have time for each other

solution... make the time to be alone together

- After a busy day, an evening run can be fun with your partner by your side.

- Enjoy some quality time in the gym. If you each want to do your own things there, meet up in the sauna or steam room afterwards and sit close.

- Go horse-riding together. You are never too old, and you'll feel muscles you didn't know you had.

Be **creative** and try to find ways to be together that don't involve food.

Learn the **rumba** (the dance of love), take up ballroom dancing or line dancing. Or just get up on the dance floor together at the next party.

Listen to **music** or take up a musical instrument together.

Be inspired by **a concert or gallery**.

Take a **romantic stroll**, hold hands and rediscover each other.

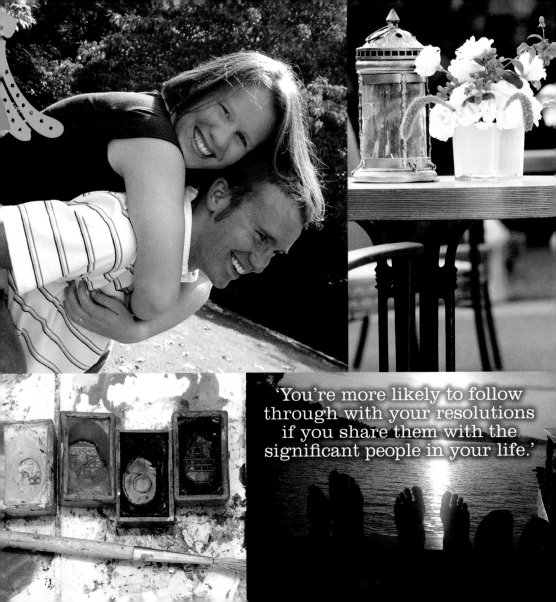

'You're more likely to follow through with your resolutions if you share them with the significant people in your life.'

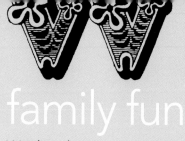

family fun

Weekends, summer evenings, Bank holidays… they're all opportunities to **bring the family together** and leave the tv and computer games behind. If food is just one part of the fun instead of the main event, it won't interfere with the day.

plan the day together

Pin up lists of possible activities in the kitchen and encourage everyone to add their own ideas. Have ideas for bad weather too so everyone doesn't just slump in front of the tv on rainy days.

fun for all

Find something that everyone can enjoy – such as a bike ride to an interesting destination. How about ice skating, roller skating or roller blading, or even indoor rock climbing? Buy everyone a pedometer and see how many miles the family can clock up in a week.

picnic food

Throw together a quick frittata with a recipe from Weight Watchers. A frittata is like a delicious quiche without the pastry.

Dig out some of the bread from inside a baguette – you can stuff it with healthy fillings and it still feels like a huge sandwich.

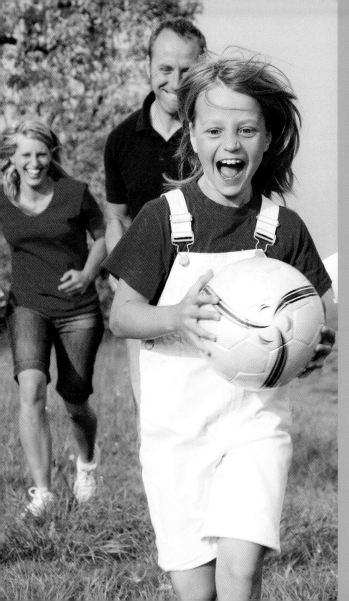

COOL DRINKS

Three-quarter fill individual bottles with water or no-added-sugar squash and freeze them. Use them as **ice packs** to keep your food cool and then you can **drink them as they thaw**. CLEVER.

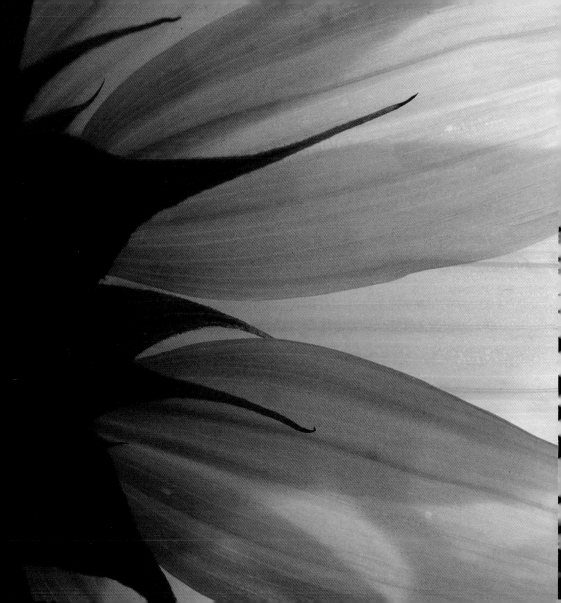

'The most wasted of all days
is one without laughter.'

ee cummings

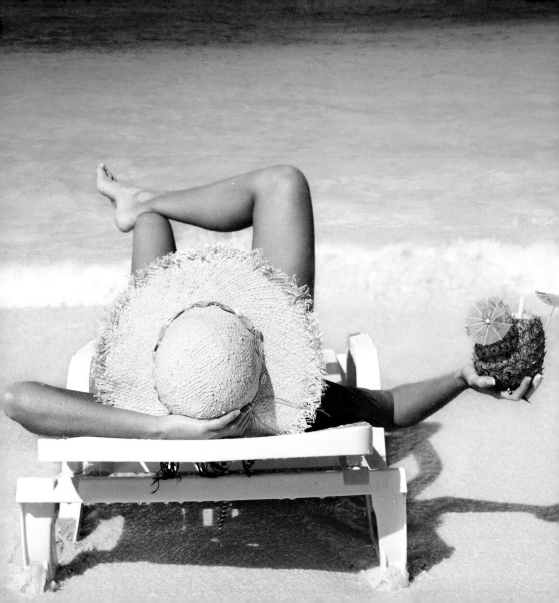

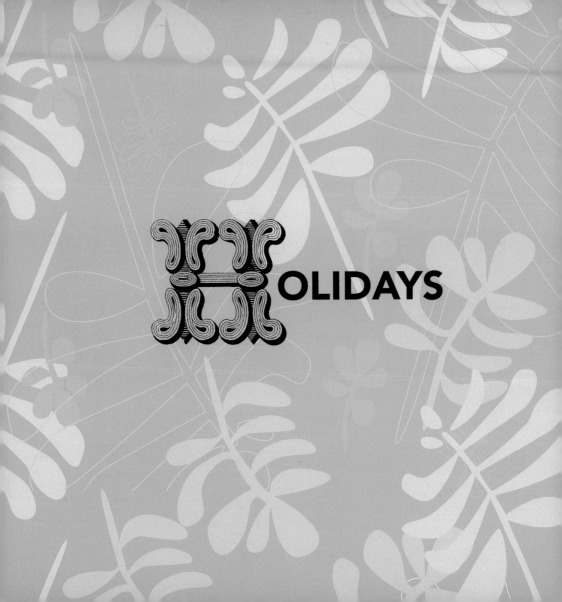

HOLIDAYS

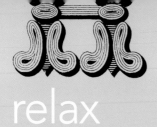

relax

problem... you really need a break but want to stick to your food plan

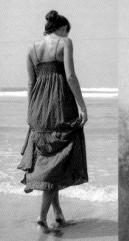

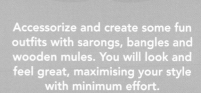

solution... stay in the 'eat wisely' frame of mind and keep active

Accessorize and create some fun outfits with sarongs, bangles and wooden mules. You will look and feel great, maximising your style with minimum effort.

♥ **Explore** Walking will clock up lots of steps and for a fab bottom workout, look for any hills and climb to the top. ♥ **Take a dip** Swimming is a great all-over body workout. ♥ **On the beach** Running and jumping in the sea can help to tone your body and it's fun. ♥ **Night life** Try out the local dance scene and keep your spirits high.

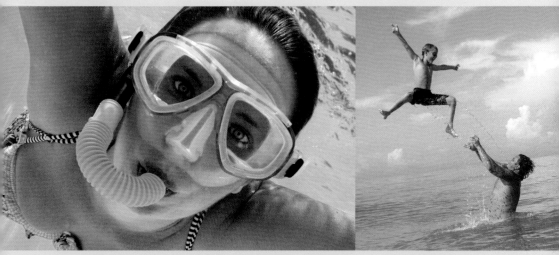

01 Don't try to lose weight on holiday – just focus on **not gaining** pounds. **02 Savour** good quality wine by the glass instead of ordering a cheap carafe. **03 Opt** for olives or crudités instead of crisps and salted nuts. **04 Forgive** yourself if you have an ice cream by the pool. Being rough on yourself is a sure-fire way to upset your weight loss goal.

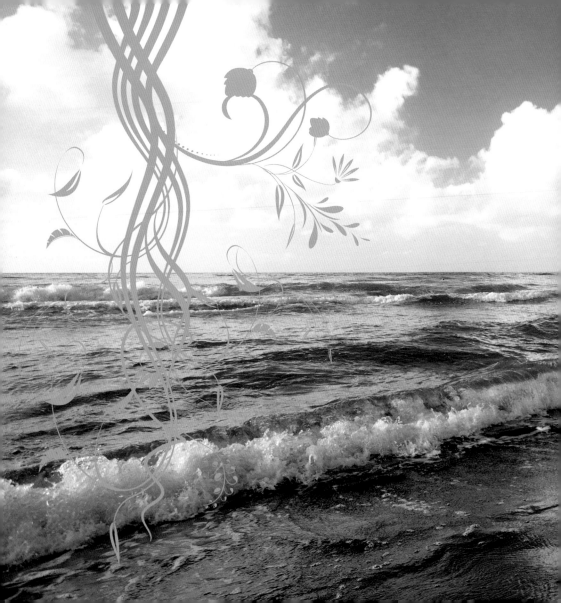

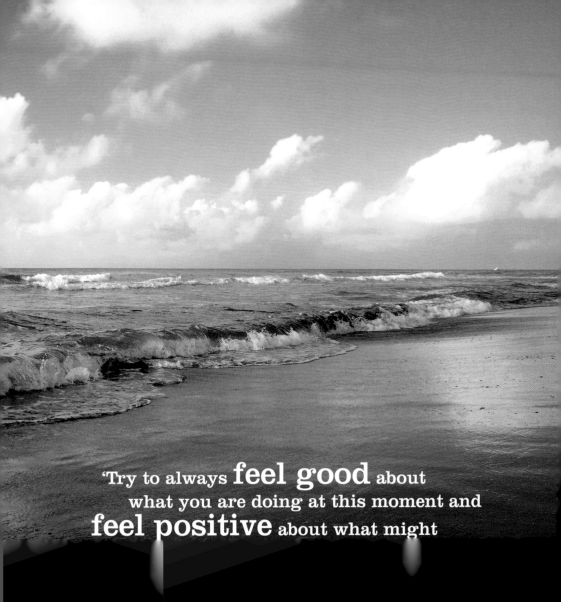

'Try to always **feel good** about what you are doing at this moment and **feel positive** about what might

post holiday blues

One minute you're **eating, drinking and laughing** in the sun. The next you're back in grey Old Blighty, possibly disappointed by any **holiday weight gain** and facing the prospect of oncoming colder weather. It's enough to make anyone give up their weight loss resolve.

...top tips to get back on track...

Be realistic Even if you did overdo it on holiday, it doesn't mean you've blown it. Accept the setbacks – some days will be easier than others. You may even find that you help yourself unconsciously by automatically reducing your intake as your holiday winds down.

Pre-arrange an exercise time You'll stick to a regime if you schedule exercise ahead. Try to get in 30 minutes almost every day. Sign up for a charity walk or run to keep to the plan.

Don't deprive yourself Focus on what you're going to eat rather than what you're not going to eat. It helps you to stick to healthy eating habits. So don't skip a nutritious, fibre-rich breakfast – it can help to prevent overeating later.

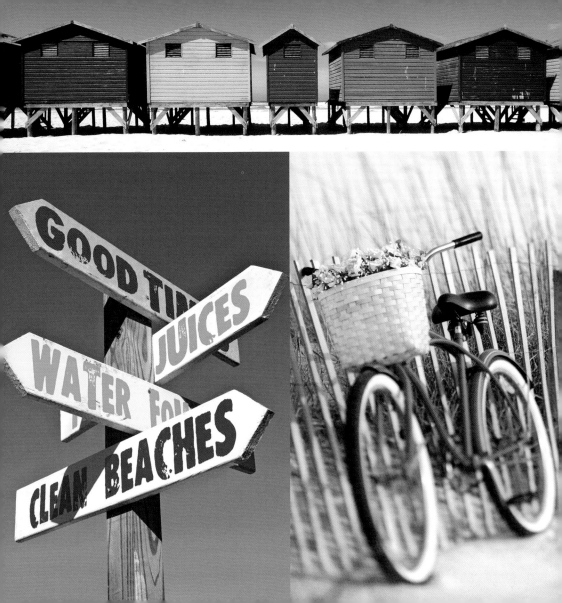

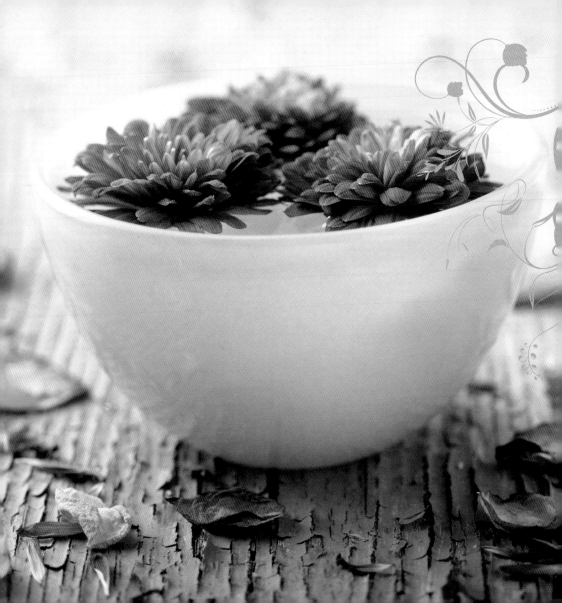

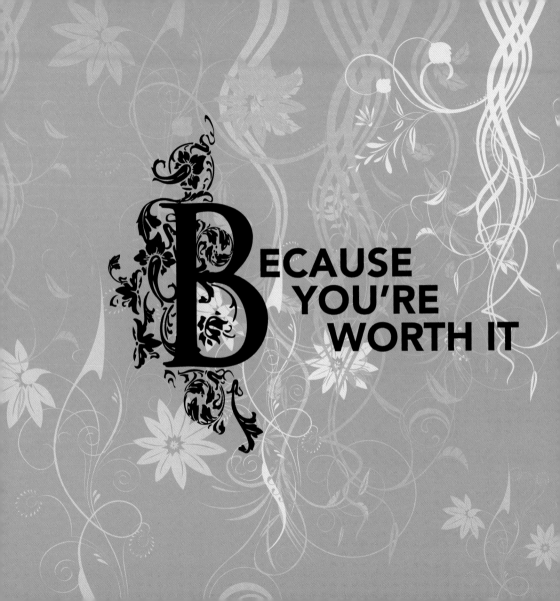

BECAUSE YOU'RE WORTH IT

mocktails & cocktails

problem... you can't remember the last time you really treated yourself

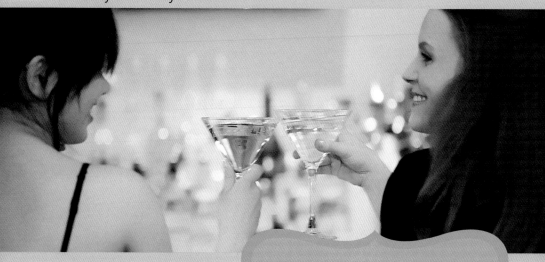

solution... a little of what you fancy does you good, so invite some friends, mix some mocktails or cocktails and **have some fun**

One way to stay in the party mood, without worrying about what you're drinking, is to enjoy some 'mocktails' – non-alcoholic versions of some old favourites.

mocktails

SHIRLEY TEMPLE Pour a splash of grenadine over a tall glass of 250ml diet Sprite.

VIRGIN MARY Mix 250ml tomato juice with a dash each of Worcestershire sauce, tabasco, salt and pepper. Add a splash of lime juice and celery salt to taste. Mix all over ice, garnish with a celery stalk and a wedge of lime.

CRANBERRY COOLER Combine 100ml cranberry juice with a splash of soda water in a highball glass. Garnish with a wedge of lime.

cocktails

BELLINI Fill a champagne flute ¼ full with fresh peach juice and add ¾ flute chilled champagne. Or try prosecco for lower alcohol content.

MIMOSA Fill a champagne flute ¼ full with fresh orange juice, then top with ¾ flute chilled champagne.

COSMOPOLITAN Shake together 1 measure vodka, ½ measure Cointreau, a splash of lime juice, 100ml cranberry juice and strain into a chilled cocktail glass.

…or just have a fabulous flute of champagne.

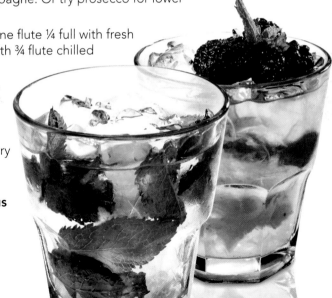

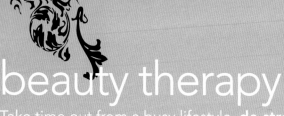

beauty therapy

Take time out from a busy lifestyle, **de-stress** your body and mind and enjoy a new you.

...luxuriate in some 'me time'...

Home spa Spending time on yourself with a home spa treatment or facial set can boost your mood and make you feel pampered.

Aromatherapy Essential oils can do wonders for emotional rejuvenation. Add 7 or 8 drops of any of the following: chamomile, rose, orange, lavender, sandalwood, ylang ylang, in any combination, to a hot, steamy bath and let those blues float away.

Get to know your skin Have your skin assessed to discover the best cleansing routine for you. Arrange a skin diagnosis before a facial to get the best products for your skin type.

Hair styling If you're getting ready for a night out, style your hair differently – with hair straighteners or curling tongs to enjoy straight or curly styles – whatever makes you feel special.

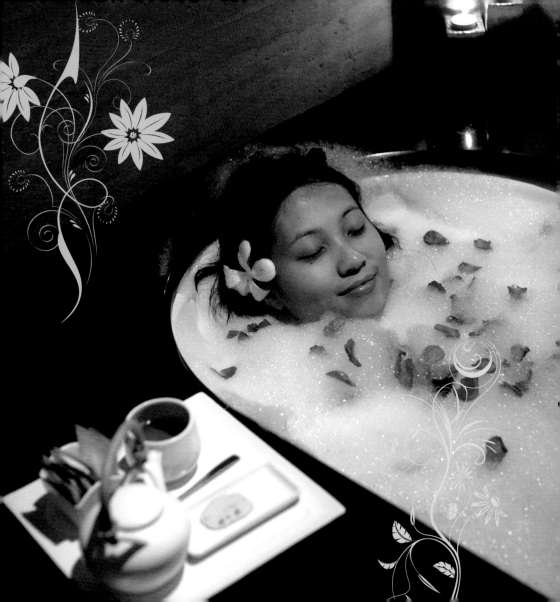

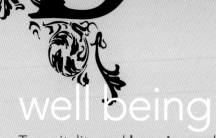

well being

True vitality and **happiness** don't come from just a few bubble baths and a couple of **early nights**. Take care of yourself and **put yourself first**, for what may be the first time in your life. You'll find the rewards are limitless so here's where to start.

Laughter A good laugh is a great tonic. Buy a joke book, go to a comedy club, rent a funny movie. The best laughter often happens with girlfriends so make an effort to meet up for coffee or go for a walk.

Sit up straight Look at your posture. Could it be improved? Maybe a course of Pilates would help. Good posture could drastically improve your appearance.

Do what you like Take time every day to do something simple that you thoroughly enjoy.

Get a social life Get out and about more – meet new people and transform your social life. Psychologists have discovered that if you put yourself first on a weight loss journey and create a balanced lifestyle, you'll have a better chance of success.

learn from the past

What's worked well for you in the past with your weight loss? If you've made mistakes in previous weight loss attempts, think of them as insights into what you need to change this time round.

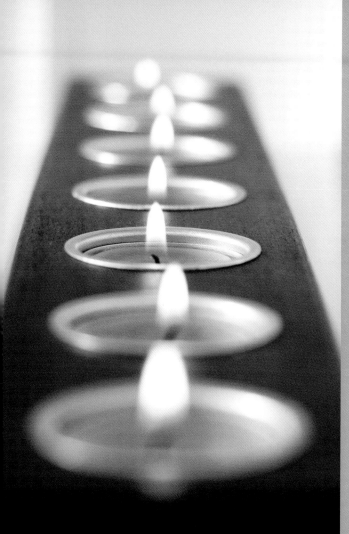

CHANGE YOUR VIEWPOINT

Stop thinking of what you're doing now as losing weight, and see it more as **eating gorgeous, healthy food**. If exercise is something you'd rather avoid, think of it as **'being active'**, **'moving more'** or **'leading an active lifestyle'**.

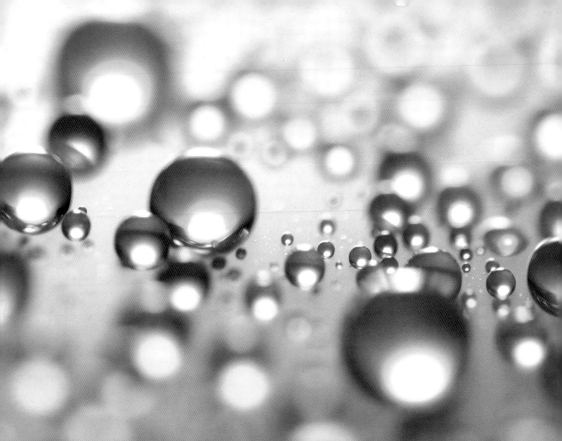

'When you **love yourself**, you start enjoying life. Break your **goals** into small, achievable ones, and **reward yourself** along the way.'

Bethany Teachman, psychologist

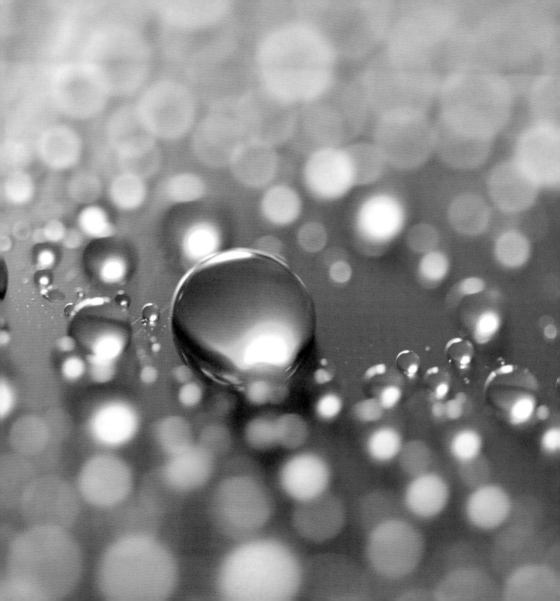

get a boost from getting active

Take control of stress with activity and do something great for your body at the same time.

Get high Step outside for your workout – it can have a very positive impact on the mind and give you that 'happy to be alive' feeling.

In the zone Being in the aerobic exercise zone (where you are breathless but still able to recite your address) causes your body to release endorphins or 'happy hormones' and create the 'runner's high' that regular exercisers are said to enjoy.

Take your best shot A boxing class or boxing circuit is a really fun way to get fit and de-stress. If you are suffering from pent-up emotions or stifled anger and stress, the physical action of punching and hitting your boxing partner's boxing pads or a punch bag can be a fantastic release.

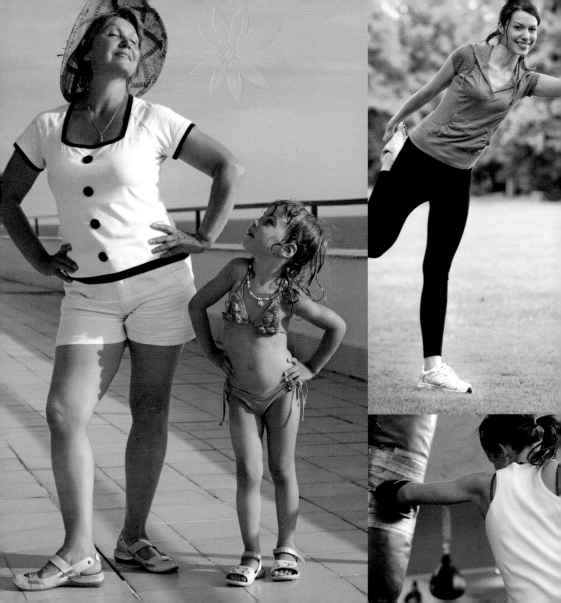

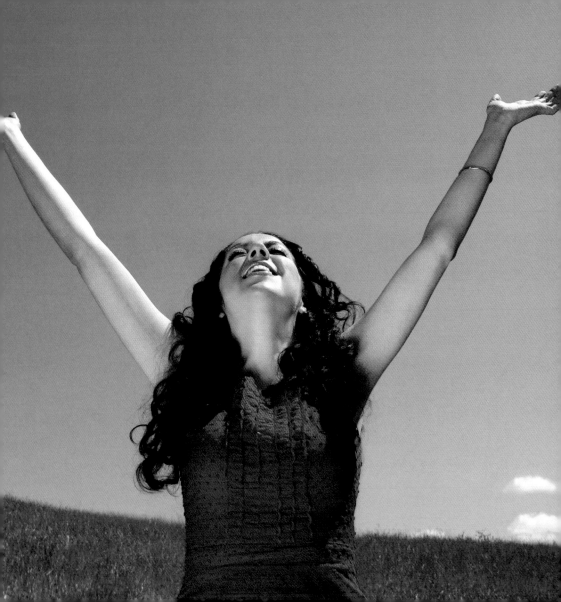

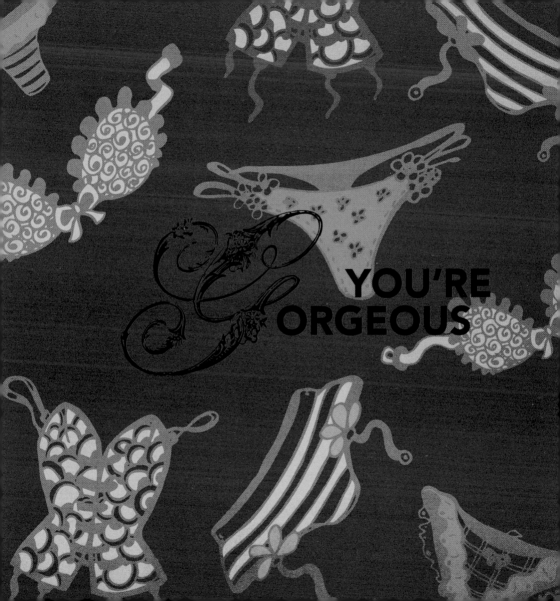

YOU'RE
GORGEOUS

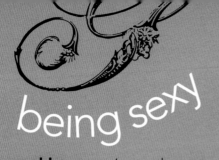

being sexy

problem... you're on the verge of quitting your weight loss plan

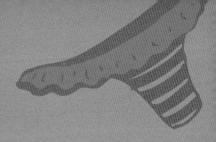

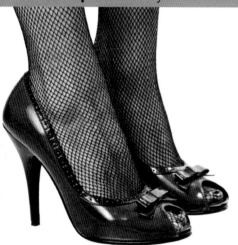

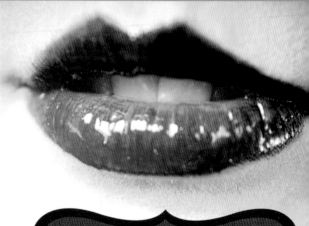

WAIT!

solution... think about what a smaller dress size can do for your sex life

Frequent lovemaking can help us lose weight, which can improve our self-esteem and physical prowess, which can then lead to more sex. It's a pretty wonderful cycle to get caught up in.

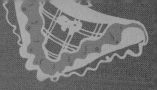

♥ Exercise helps you to stay **flexible**, which means you can assume more sexual positions than you might have otherwise. ♥ *Variety is the spice of a good sex life.* ♥ When you're at a healthy weight and in good aerobic condition, you may be able to have sex for longer and exert yourself better.

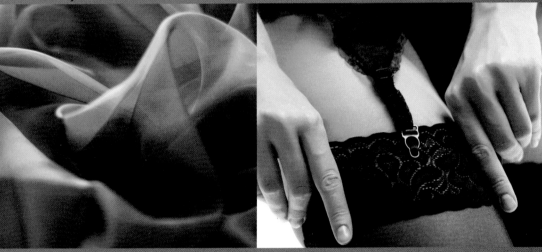

01 As you lose weight and get into better shape, you look and feel better. The result? You'll be more prone to take the initiative and feel more enthusiastic. **02** Feeling strong and virile can be an excellent aphrodisiac. **03** Being in good shape gives you more energy so you're likely to have sex more often.

you deserve to look good

Take time to make yourself **feel beautiful** and get the **confidence** you need to step out in style. Feeling good about yourself is a surefire **way to success**.

Luscious lips For an instant pout, wear clear lip gloss to create a natural look.

Eye-catching To accentuate your eyes, try a good lengthening and defining mascara, using one or two coats to customise your lashes and really make them stand out.

Rosy cheeks A quick dusting of a tinted blush brings a healthy glow to cheek bones.

Revitalised hair To get maximum volume into your hair, spritz a good lifting spray into the roots when almost dry, wrap sections of hair around a large roller, blast with cool air and wait 10 minutes before removing.

Make-up bag MOT 'Out with the old and in with the new' – make this your make-up motto. Keep your make-up tools clean and renew your make-up regularly.

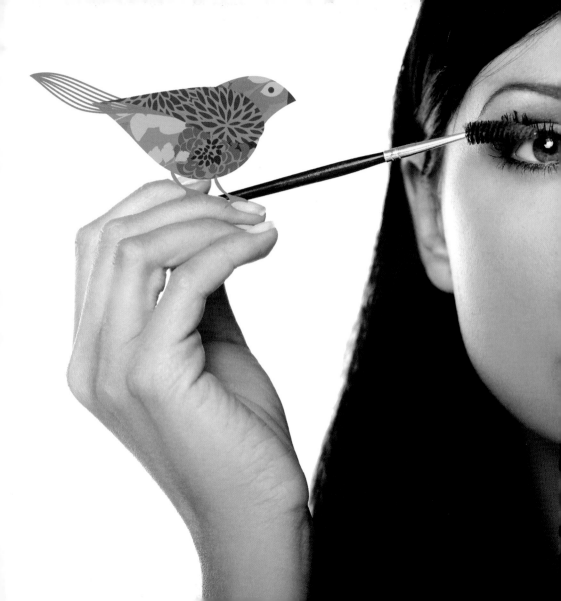

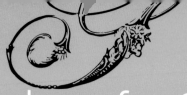

dress for SUCCESS

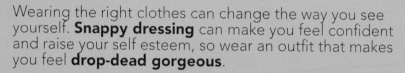

Wearing the right clothes can change the way you see yourself. **Snappy dressing** can make you feel confident and raise your self esteem, so wear an outfit that makes you feel **drop-dead gorgeous**.

take the goddess test

When you try something on, ask yourself: 'Does this make me feel like a goddess?' Whether it's a pair of black trousers, a plain white t-shirt, or a cocktail dress – do you really feel fantastic wearing that piece of clothing?

slimming style

Wearing black is always a great option – it's elegant and can create a slimming silhouette. Inject colour with scarves, handbags and fantastic boots or shoes but avoid too much colour contrast. Don't break the flow of the eye from the shoulder to the floor and you'll get a longer and leaner body line.

limit comfort clothes

Limit yourself to no more than two 'TV' jumpers. Much more flattering are slim-fitting and tailored jerseys or tops. They give you a much sleeker and confident look, and will make you feel that way too.

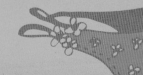

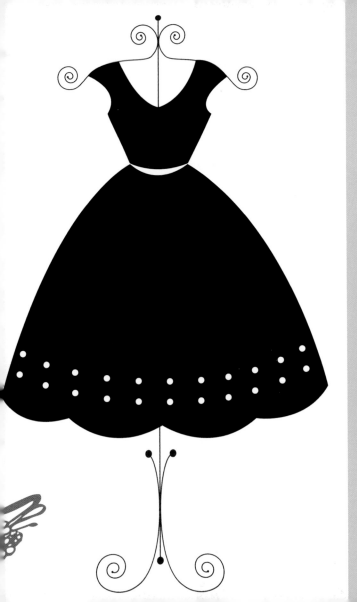

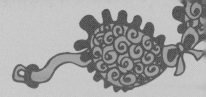

ONLY WEAR SEXY KNICKERS

Wearing gorgeous underwear is a great foundation for **looking and feeling fantastic**. It's about recognizing your value, and being kind to yourself **because you're worth it**.

'THINK BEAUTIFUL
Walk, talk and relate as though
you're a **beautiful gazelle**…

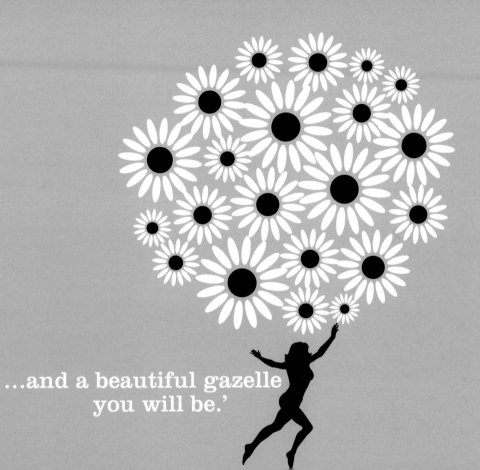

'...and a beautiful gazelle
you will be.'

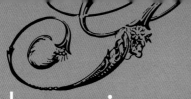

happiness, the beauty within

To look your very best, beauty needs to be on the inside too.

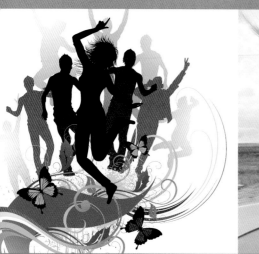

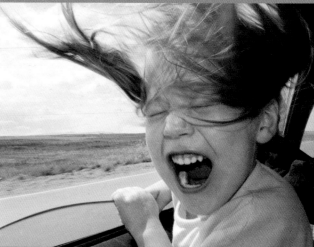

When you believe in yourself, you radiate a positive energy that people find irresistible...

...so get the positive vibe.

'Get rid of 'shoulds' and 'oughts' – set yourself free to enjoy the moment.'

Take hold of happiness now

What could you do today to 'up' your happiness quota? **01 Join** an art class. **02 Write** to an old friend. **03 Learn** a new recipe. **04 Start** a book club. **05 Clean out** a cupboard and **give** some things away to charity.

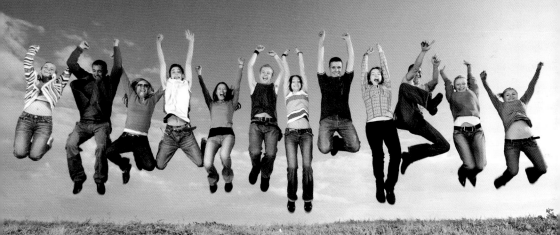

- ♥ Replace every negative thought with a **positive** one. Instead of 'I hate my hips', try 'I really like my eyes'.
- ♥ Say '**thank you**' to compliments, instead of putting yourself down in response.
- ♥ If you see an **opportunity**, train yourself to say 'yes' first and then deal with the details afterwards.

Acknowledgements

Text sources

All text throughout the book is from weightwatchers.co.uk, except where indicated below.

pages 28–29: K Miller-Kovach, *Healthy Parent, Healthy Child.* London, 2009.

pages 62–63: Attributed to ee cummings.

pages 68–69: "Everybody loves a winner", *Weight Watchers Magazine* (August 2009), page 98.

Picture credits

All cover images from Shutterstock except the handbag, drawn by Fiona Andreanelli.

All other images throughout the book from Shutterstock except where indicated below.

iStock: pages 13, 15 (top right), 18 (right), 19, 21, 26 (left), 34 (left), 35, 36–37, 39, 40, 43, 45, 47, 48, 50, 55, 59 (top left), 74, 83 (bottom right), 84, 86, 91, 94 (left) and 95.

Francine Lawrence, pages 28–29